I0791485

HOW TO REDUCE YOUR WEIGHT & KEEP IT OFF

A Simple Solution to your Weight Problem

J. MAURICE ROBERTS

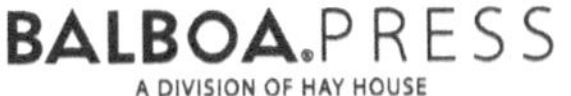

Balboa Press books may be ordered through booksellers or by contacting:

Balboa Press
A Division of Hay House
1663 Liberty Drive
Bloomington, IN 47403
www.balboapress.co.uk
UK TFN: 0800 0148647 (Toll Free inside the UK)
UK Local: 02036 956325 (+44 20 3695 6325 from outside the UK)

Print information available on the last page.

ISBN: 978-1-9822-8183-0 (sc)
ISBN: 978-1-9822-8184-7 (e)

Balboa Press rev. date: 07/17/2020

ACKNOWLEDGEMENTS

This manual would not have been possible without the support and sound advice of friends and colleagues, some of whom are engaged in the "Healing" Profession.To that end, I especially extend my thanks and gratitude to:

Dr. Elizabeth Muir. GP & Senior Clinical Lecturer.
Dr. Rory Read. GP
Dermot O'Gorman – Chiropractor (Specialising in the McTimoney Technique.
Mrs. Jill Evans and Mrs Liz. Hudson for their help in the layout and formatting of this "Road Map", showing the way to a successful outcome.
Mrs Margaret Grant for ensuring the "Naaman Paradox" was easily digestible.

To the many others who have heard my thoughts and challenges and have in countless ways helped and inspired me to persevere and write this Solution to the Weight Control problem experienced by so many.

We are all shaped in some way by the people we associate with, the people we meet, the books we read, the stories we hear, the people we are inspired by, and who become our mentors.

These are just some of the people who have inspired me.

Dr Deepak Chopra M.D. – Father Anthony de Mello. SJ - Dr Wayne Dyer. Psychotherapist – Napoleon Hill, author –Og Mandino- Bob Proctor – Tony Robbins – Jim Rohn – Brian Tracy.

N.B. The views and suggestions in this guide are those of the author.

DEDICATION

To Anne, my lovely wife of 40 years, before she was taken prematurely from me.

She was always my mentor and my guide, helping me to see the best in everyone and providing a positive perspective, in even the darkest of situations we experienced on 'Life's Journey". The day we met was the day my Life was changed and enriched forever. Sometimes people mistook her gentleness and humility as weakness, till they experienced the deep spiritual reservoirs from which she drew her strength.

To my children: Christopher, John, Caroline, Jeremy and Charlotte. For the many things I learned from them, albeit, often reluctantly. Too often I came from the position of "I know what is best". Humility is not an easy lesson to learn, but they taught me graciously.

To my Grandchildren: Sallyanne, Rebecca, Sam, Jack, Annie, Joshua Isabella, Chaya. - the next generation to keep me on track and to remind me that "out of the mouths ...." comes unfettered wisdom, if we are open to receive. The questions they asked, often left me feeling, "Wow! Now why didn't I think of that"?

To my two brothers, and sister, Den, Merle, and Fred. For the growing up together – for the many activities and games we shared – the competitiveness – the humour – the antics involved in sibling rivalry. Foundations laid well.

To my Mum, Caroline and Dad John. Mum, gentle and caring but taken too soon. Dad, who left brief glimpses of himself before he died when I was nine years old.

To the folks I know, all written in a book

And every year at Christmas time, I go and take a look.

For each name stands for someone who has touched my life, sometime?

I really feel that I'm composed, of each remembered name

And my life is so much better, than it was before they came

To all those many people who are sick to death of their weight issues and whom I hope and pray will be helped by my "Solutions"

PREPARATION BEFORE THE ADVENTURE BEGINS

It's been said countless times that we spend more time, thought and research planning a holiday or a vacation than we spend on planning and shaping our lives. Is that you?

Holidays last a couple or a few weeks, while OUR LIVES are longer and much more important.

Life, is like a 'cuppa'; it's how we make it". I like my tea hot, strong, a dash of milk, and some sugar. I'm a 'Mil' person – "milk in last". The tea aficionados say pour boiling water – leave to brew.

Some just wave the bag, in and out to colour the water – some have milk in the cup, then add boiling water; some add mint, ginger, or lemon. Coffee drinkers like it white – black – sugar – no sugar – real or instant. Some instant drinkers almost count the grains.

A Choice – a Conscious Decision about a mundane daily routine.

Character is formed the same way. Suddenly you are an artist creating a sculpture, which reflects the real you. Character, doesn't just happen, any more than a chisel can create a work of art without the artists guiding hand.

Character is not something we were born with. It is the result of hundreds of choices and decisions.

You are the artist, sculpting the you, you aim to be.

There are some people who leave you feeling good no matter the circumstances. There are others who drag you down. What have you the artist created? Which category do you fall into?

Serious Question to ask yourself and let the honest answers emerge.

We have to look inside; often step outside comfort zones – sometimes into the unknown.

VISION TAKES COURAGE AND COMMITMENT

So, before we start let me share a few thoughts with you.

- When we were children, we grew up being told that we should do what our parents and authority figures told us to do and accept, and not question or challenge anything. We now know that some of the problems in society today are as a direct result of erroneous programming, albeit, sometimes that was done with loving intentions.
- I am recommending a process that you take on board, but I'm also suggesting you think about it and challenge the concepts, before you accept them for yourself. I want you to accept, for yourself, the validity of my methods for helping you achieve success, and perhaps more importantly, grow as a person.
- As you progress, I would urge you to read each quotation and then take time to see or hear what it is saying to you. (I know what each one is saying to me). This is an important 'marker' on the road to your change.

Here, you have an opportunity to take control, and my hope is that as we travel together, I will help you to SUCCEED.

Before starting anything, whether it's a journey or a project we generally make some preparations; jot down steps to take, list things we will need. Imagine asking a builder to build your dream home, without providing the architect's drawings

Embarking on this solution to your weight problem is no different, so here are some thoughts to ponder on.

The process is set down as steps to take. Steps can sometimes be in a straight line, sometimes random. In one situation you might be walking, following steps leading you along a path from A to B. In other situations, such as dancing, your steps could be forwards – backwards – sideways and so on.

1. Certainly, this programme is organised in a way, which allows you to be doing more than one suggestion at a time, to help you to achieve success more speedily. Walk or Dance as the occasion requires. Have fun"

2. My suggestion is that you might prefer to have a quick 'jog' through before you start, so you have an idea of the layout. Almost like a rambler having a quick look at his ordinance survey map before he sets out, as this gives him an inkling of what lies ahead.

3. You will soon see that I believe life provides different views, depending on which perspective you are looking from. I call these "THE FLIP SIDE of LIFE". With an 'up' there is a 'down'; 'in' has an 'out'; 'front' has a 'back' and so on. There is always another perspective.

4. Greek and Roman scholars believed, "the question is more important than the answer." If you do not ask the right question, you will never get the right answer.

There is a story to illustrate what I am getting at —
you will find it at the end of our "Preparation Notes".
I'm sure it will make you smile.

5. There are "Sayings" sprinkled throughout this manual
    to "Weight Reduction and Control" and a healthier
    LIFE. They serve a purpose.

    Please take time to look, to read, and to let them
    "speak" to you – "resonate" within you, and to laugh.
    The quotations have a purpose.

    Find the meaning for you. What do they say
    to you?

6. As we grew up as children, we were told, by our parents
    and other authority figures, to accept statements
    without question. We no longer have that restriction,
    so, by all means challenge thoughts and suggestions as
    they resonate within you. If need be, check statements
    out, BUT with this caution. "Do not use it as an
    excuse to opt / cop out and do nothing."

The ideas and suggestions DO WORK.
The question always is, **"Will you work them"?**

**ACTION – ACTION – ACTION –ACTION – ACTION –
ACTION** is KEY. Write your notes in a journal or note book.

Here is a poem which should give you pause for thought

"The Road Not Taken"
Robert Frost. (1874-1963) American poet

Two Roads diverged in a yellow wood,
And, sorry I could not travel both
And be one traveller, long I stood
And looked down one as far as I could
To where it bent in the undergrowth;
Then took the other, just as fair,
And having perhaps the better claim
Because it was grassy and wanted wear;
Though as for that the passing there
Had worn them really about the same

And both that morning equally lay
In leaves no step had trodden black.
Oh, I kept the first for another day!
Yet knowing, how way leads on to way,
I doubted if I should ever come back.

I shall be telling this with a sigh
Somewhere ages and ages hence:
Two roads diverged in a wood, and I -
I took the one less travelled by,
And that has made all the difference

THE SHOP AROUND THE CORNER – OR – THE CORNER SHOP

There is always one of those.

In days gone by there were many more of the family shops and no doubt there still are such shops. However, these days, there are also the huge Supermarkets open 24 hours– with the neon sign which says: - **OPEN ALL HOURS.**

Let's say you want to nip out for a new face. Not so farfetched, if you think about it. Every day, you choose the face you carry around with you.

You have thought about it and chosen the face you present to the world.

Think of the decisions you have made, and some of the characteristics you have opted for.

Men: Clean shaven – full beard or goatee – full moustache or just covering the upper lip – long hair – short - crew cut –short or long sideburns - no hair -earrings, - nose rings – tattoos visible or hidden etc.

Women: Long hair – short hair - styled – hanging loose - earrings – nose rings – tattoos visible or hidden - make-up – no make- up – shade of lipstick etc.

EVERY DAY- We make a very conscious decision as to how we look, facially. We make a choice

Yet – and isn't it strange, that we do not give as much attention to the rest of ourselves:

Physically   Mentally   Spiritually.

The size and shape of our bodies will often dictate the style and colour of the clothes we wear. We make conscious decisions about how we dress: the style – the colours – often to camouflage the size and shape of our bodies, while wishing we could wear something different.

It's like going into the "FACE SHOP" only, and ignoring the rest of the features that make up the real you!

Let's go shopping! Have you got your list or are you just going to see what catches your eye?

OK! You have your selection, from the "Head & Face" Department.

Now is the time to select the Mind — Body and — Spirit

The YOU – you Aspire to BE!

Getting Started is the key: Momentum then takes over

Begin >>>>>>>>> Every Beginner is A WINNER!

To achieve success you must make a start!

It doesn't matter how you get started. So long as you get started!

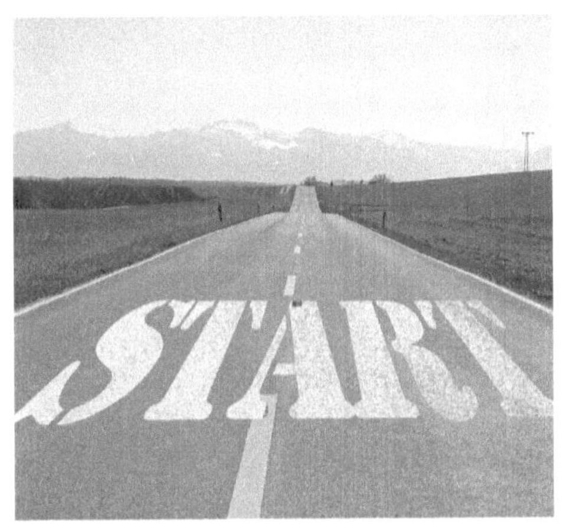

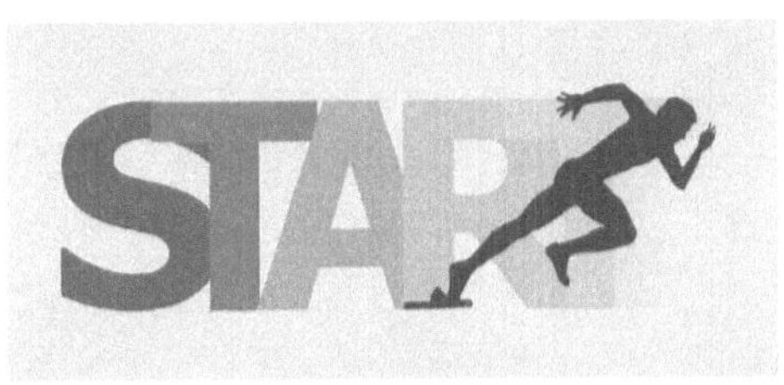

Just get STARTED

INTRODUCTION

"LET ME BE YOUR GUIDE AND MENTOR"!

As a therapist and counsellor, I have worked with people of different ages, shapes and sizes and with a host of differing problems. The learning, the "AHA" moment for them, has been the realisation that almost all problems stem from the same cause – negative thoughts and programmes buried in our subconscious mind.

Our minds are like computers. Whether you use a computer or not, virtually everyone will have some knowledge of how a computer works, and the impact it has in, and, on our daily lives.

Load the wrong programme and you will never get the result that you are hoping to achieve.

Our language is dotted with clichés and, over-used, they become a source of irritation. I'm going to share one with you.

G.I.G.O. "Garbage in – Garbage out".

When you throw your rubbish in the dustbin, or trash in the trash can, what would you expect to see if you tipped the bin or can over? Gold bars? Now, that would be wonderful, wouldn't it? But – not likely to happen?

Einstein had this to say, "Doing exactly the same thing tomorrow as you have done today and then expecting a different outcome is the first sign of insanity"!

The message, clear, simple and unambiguous is this, "When we break our patterns new worlds emerge". So my suggestion is for you to break some patterns and let your new world emerge.

In this journey I will offer suggestions to change your behaviour, eat better, eliminate the fixation with food, speed up your metabolism and help you to feel terrific about yourself.

Neither I, nor any other therapist, rely on 'magic wands'. I won't be waving a magic wand, but work with me and the end result is, often, magical.

I will work with what you bring to the process. The answers and the solutions are already within you. You have a decision to make.

Do you want to be slimmer? Yes or No?

Will you do what needs to be done? Patterns will have to be broken. Are you ready to do that? **If the answer, genuinely, is "Yes", let's continue.**

If the answer is "No", then quite bluntly, pass this on and don't waste your precious time, for life and time are truly precious. The sad fact of life is that there are people who will say, "It didn't work" and tell others that. When asked the question, "What didn't work"? you discover that they didn't take the steps to change.

If you have decided to say, "YES", then read on.

There is no magic wand that eliminates participation in the change process!

By saying "YES", we have a pact – you and I! You are promising commitment to the process and the exciting journey ahead and I have promised to show you the way.

I know the process works!

First, let's play a little game.

NB: Read this next paragraph before you play!!! Why? Because you can't read with your eyes closed!!!!!! Ha, Ha, Ha. Take a moment now.

Close your eyes and breathe easily; Now, in your mind's eye, see yourself as you want to be; relax and enjoy the vision of the NEW you. What colour clothes are you wearing? Are they your favourite colour? SMILE! Done that? OK. Open your eyes. Keep the SMILE, and remember the "vision" of the new you and enjoy the experience.

Now Play the Game. Then PLAY IT AGAIN

Have fun – enjoy the journey! **Life is not "a Sentence" to be served**

It's an exciting Adventure to be LIVED

The Adventure begins!

PROLOGUE

THE NAAMAN PARADOX!

I know of a psychiatrist, whose first question to a client is, "Do you believe in the Scriptures"? Whether the answer is "Yes" or "No", his response is the same.

"Good! Read this passage from Scripture", and he would give them a passage to read. Remember, the Bible is a special book containing solutions., But give it the LABEL- "BIBLE" and sometimes people do not open the BOOK.!!

One of my many mentors, Jim Rohn, once described the Bible as 'a collection of stories' that were either examples or warnings, and then went on to ask, "Would you want your life story to be in there as an example or a warning?"

At this point you are probably wondering where I'm going with this? Be patient and all will be revealed.

Why is it that we humans are so suspicious of simple solutions, believing, that for a solution to be effective, it has to be complicated and difficult to implement?

The solutions I am going to reveal to you, to achieve weight control, are simple, so you might be tempted to ignore and even denigrate them. **If you do so, you do yourself a dis-service**

I said 'Simple'. Easy? Well! That's for you to decide!

If someone offered you a gold nugget or a diamond, wrapped in some tissue paper rather than in a jeweller's box, would you accept or refuse?

Refusal, of this solution, would be tantamount to shooting the messenger who is bringing you a simple but effective weight control solution!

One of the Bible's most instructive moments is:
The Story of Naaman. (Paraphrased below).

"Naaman, Captain of the King of Aram's army was a great and honourable man and admired by the King, because by him, he had won many victories over his enemies. He was a very brave man – but, he was a leper."

It is ironic that despite Naaman's strength and success, in the eyes of Israel and most of the ancient world, his disease of leprosy was associated with un-cleanliness, and that fact completely eclipsed his greatness!

When Naaman heard, from a captive slave, that there was, in Samaria, a prophet of God who reputedly could cure him of his dread disease, he journeyed to the house of the Prophet Elisha. There, Naaman sought healing from his leprosy at the hand of the Prophet.

The Scriptures say, that in response to Naaman's request, Elisha sent a messenger out, saying "Go and wash in the Jordan seven times and you will be cured".

The act that would bring about Naaman's healing, immersing himself in the Jordan River seven times – was so un-dramatic, that Naaman, oblivious to the symbolic reference to the seven day quarantine required of a leper in Israel and oblivious also to the importance of humility, obedience, and faith, was offended and refused to comply.

The story continues: "Naaman was angry, and went away, saying, "I thought, he will at least come out to see me, and stand, and call on the name of his God, and lay his hand over the place, and cure the leprosy".

"Are not Abana and Pharpar, rivers of Damascus, better than all the waters of Israel? May I not wash in them, and be clean? So he turned and went away in a rage."

Naaman seems to have been angered on two counts: first, that Elisha would communicate with him through a mere servant rather than honouring him with a personal response; and second, that the promised cure should involve an action on Naaman's part, a simple action at that, rather than a dramatic miracle at the hand of the prophet.

The scriptures say that following his indignant refusal, Naaman's own servants convinced him to return. His servants came and said to him, "Sir, if the prophet had asked you to do some great thing, wouldn't you have done it? Why not then when he says, "Wash, and be clean", will you not do it? Then Naamam went down, and dipped himself seven times in the Jordan, according to the instructions of the man of God, and he was cured.

01

Just to remind you of what I asked you at the start:

Why is it that we humans are so suspicious of the simple solutions, believing that for a solution to be effective, it has to be complicated and difficult to implement?

Step 1- Cause and Effect and Myths about Dieting

Medical conditions apart, there will always be fat and obese people. Maybe, they have no desire to change. But that is not you, or you would not be reading this.

Whether your main goal is to reduce weight, lead a healthier lifestyle, feel really happy with your body or just be able to control your eating habits, this system is designed for you. But the choice is yours. **"To do or not to do! TO BE- - or not to be - The you, you want to be"**.

In the Star Wars film, Yoda says:

"There is no trying. There is only DO — or don't do".

Let me repeat that: "There is only "DO" -------- or "DON'T DO"

Either way you will get a result.

The problem with "Trying" is that you are leaving yourself a loop hole – an open back door – an escape route. I have been in the situation where someone has asked me to do something and my response has been, "I'll try"!

Then, when asked why I haven't done whatever I said I would try to do, my answer has been:-

"I didn't say I'd do it. I said I'd try"! If that isn't a cop - out!'

Ever been there?

There is no trying. There is only DO or don't do".

Read the poem below; then get a notebook and write your answers to the questions below. Be honest with yourself. If you aren't, you are only cheating yourself!

Have you got your notebook ready?
What do you want to look like?
What are you prepared to do, to achieve success?
What size are you?
What size do you want to be?
What colour are you wearing?
What colours would you like to wear?
Why do you want to embark on this journey of change?
When would you like to be the YOU, you envisage?
How are you going to achieve this goal of yours?
Where will you celebrate each achievement and with Whom?
Who are you doing this for?
If you are not as you would like to be, there must be reasons. Answering the questions will help you chart your

course. Before you start your adventure you should know two things. Where the start line is and Where the finish line is.

That established, you will have your goal in sight.

Take a moment: close your eyes- picture yourself as the "YOU - YOU want to be".

There are a few patterns that seem to be common among people who wish to reduce and control their weight.

- Dieting - almost obsessively so and often switching from one dieting regime to another and then yet another?
- Dieting - suggests forbidden foods, restrictions, calorie counting, and, watching, watching, watching! This possibly causes one to focus on what one cannot have.

Have you heard the expression: "It's like watching paint dry." There must be better things to watch, than watching the scales so frequently. Why not watch nature and let the birds, bees, trees, flowers work their magic within you.

Yes! People do lose weight, but then find after a while that they are back where they started, or that all the joy has been squeezed out of the pleasure of eating.

Have you been there?

There is an interesting concept to be considered about the choice of words.

If we **lose** something our normal reaction is to attempt to find it. The body is no different, governed as it is by the brain.

Be aware of your choice of words

Dieting, generally, has connotations, because of the way the body processes the deprivation and demand for food.

The more diets that people try and fail at, the more they suffer a sense of failure and subsequent loss of self-esteem.

It seems, that reducing people's diets to a state of semi-starvation, often produces symptoms of irritability, loss of endurance and energy and obsessive behaviour about food, including, but not restricted to, lying, stealing and hoarding.

Depriving the body of food seems to be the least attractive way to reduce weight. So, the suggestion here is, that if what you have been doing isn't working, there has to be another way.

Changing your mind-set --------- is the way forward.

Emotional eating is generally considered to be the main cause of obesity. After the yo-yo of dieting regimes.

Often people eat because they are bored, lonely, unhappy, with time on their hands, tired or stressed, and for many other emotional reasons, which have nothing to do with hunger – physical hunger.

Then, because, very often, they are on their own, they go for the nibbles and binge on Crisps – Chocolate bars etc., which they know are not good for them. A bingeing habit is formed and, without thinking, they eat what they know is not good for them.

I remember vividly, one client of mine who was very much in this mould. Simply getting him to focus on getting him out of the house and pursuing a desired activity solved his problem

There is an alternative. While you are learning to change your mind set and the habit of putting something in your mouth choose a much healthier option. Eating a variety of fruits comes to mind.

If you eat because of emotional hunger, your body will never feel physical satisfaction because of your food intake.

Imagine this:

You pull into a petrol station because you need fuel, but instead of going to the pumps you go across the forecourt and fill your tyres with air!

So let me repeat :-

If you eat because of emotional hunger, your body will never feel physical satisfaction because of your food intake.

Emotional hunger is never satisfied by food. It will only feel satisfied by emotional fulfilment. That makes sense, doesn't it?

That is when the little small voice may ask you, "Am I really hungry or do I just want some loving and affection and thereby change the way I feel?"

If you want to change your emotional state, no amount of food will do it, except perhaps make you physically sick.

The answer? - change your mind programme.

Very often, men and women, find their weight gain started with some traumatic incident in their lives – loss of job leading to loss of self-esteem for instance. Sometimes it may be sexual abuse, teasing or ridicule in front of others; rejection by partners or peers leading to excessive embarrassment.

Many people have grown up with eating habits that lead to weight gain.

The techniques here will help, but remember they are not intended as substitutes for professional medical assistance. If you think this could apply to you, visit your doctor or consult an appropriate professional therapist for specific treatment.

Faulty Programming. If you are carrying more weight than you want, it probably is the natural progression of your present mental programmes. It means that you have to make some changes in your life.

The lovely aspect of making changes is, that 'change generally comes bearing gifts'.

You must have heard the old saying :- Chin up Chest out!

Find your own way of changing your state: whistle a tune – sing a song – take a deep abdominal breath – do a twirl – do a handstand – jump on the spot – go for a short walk – stretch and ease your muscles, laugh out loud – whatever suits you.

IT'S YOUR LIFE

If you are ready to change your life, you have to change certain habits.

Taken from, "An autobiography in five short chapters. By Portia Nelson.

CHANGE

I walk down a street, there is a deep hole in the pavement.
I see it is there, but I fall in
I walk down the same street, there's still a deep hole in the pavement
I fall in again.
I walk down the same street and fall in again. It's a habit
I walk down the same street. I see the hole there. I walk round it.
I walk down a different street

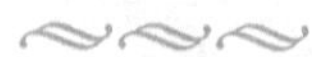

The Power of Habit

You should know me. I'm your constant companion.
I'm your greatest helper; I'm your heaviest burden.
Half the tasks you do might as well be turned over to me.
I will push you onward or drag you down to failure.
I am at your command.
Be easy with me, and I will destroy you.
Be firm with me, and I'll put the world at your feet.
Who am I? I'm Habit!

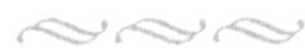

Author unknown.

What habits would you like to change? Write them down!

To change anything you have to — TAKE ACTION

Let's play another little game. When you've done with the playing, you have a choice to make. Simply decide 'do' or 'not do'.

Then take responsibility for your decision

Imagine you are standing outside your front door and it's locked. You have the key, but it is in your pocket or purse. You can leave it in your pocket or purse and stand there on the outside, or you can take the key out, insert it in the lock and let yourself in. Which option did you choose?

Here is another thought. Whatever you are doing – sitting or standing, it doesn't matter.

Now! Without getting up or taking a physical step, move to another location in the room. Unless you take action and move yourself you will remain sitting or standing wherever you are.

Action is the Key

There are a host of suggestions like these, but I'm sure you get the point.

Whatever your decision there will be consequences. Certain immutable laws govern the Universe. It doesn't matter whether we like them or not, these laws operate.

First, let's take the 'Law of Gravity'. Unless you are on the moon, if you jump off a multi-story building, yelling, "I don't believe in Gravity", you will not change the fact that you will end up in a heap as you hit the ground – thud!

Another Law is that of "Cause and Effect". You take some action, and it will produce a result. You don't take any action and that will also produce a result. That's a fact of life.

One thing I would urge you, however, is not to have any feelings of guilt should you choose not to take action. Feelings of guilt inevitably lead one to look for scapegoats, so that we can deposit the blame somewhere.

Guilt is a merry-go-round you don't want to be on. Believe me!

Whatever your decision, take responsibility for your decision and live with the consequences and move on. That's life! It's your life! ☺

But remember: **LIFE is not a sentence to be served**
Life is to be LIVED with Enthusiasm

Cause and Effect! This system works, BUT you have to be engaged in the process.

A song says: "Ready, Willing and Able"!

If you say "Yes", let's move on.

02

Step 2. The Adventure Begins

The Greeks called the beginning Alpha. We start our language with the letter A, so it seems A is a very appropriate place to start our Adventure.

Did you notice I said "Adventure" Consider it an adventure, because it conjures up so many emotions: - excitement - trepidation - risk – jubilation. I'm sure you can add your own emotions to that list. Well, you can – can't you?

Dictionaries lead us into an Aladdin's cave of language – words for all purposes and occasions. Let's explore a few. Isn't that what adventurers do? Explore!

Adventure: An unusual experience or course of events marked by excitement and suspense.

Attitude: A state of mind and way of behaving.

Awareness: Well informed, sensitive and perceptive

Action: Something done, movement, posture

Everything of substance is usually laid on firm foundations, or there is the danger of collapse. The journey you are about to embark on will be fun if you treat it as such and remember the four A's

Before you can make any changes you have to have an awareness of where you are now - or put another way, how can you change anything if you don't know that it needs to be changed, or want to change it?

Every new activity has to be learned. Repetition, Repetition, Repetition, then it becomes a habit – second nature.

Do you remember the first time you tied your shoelaces or a bow? Tough, wasn't it? You thought, 'I'll never get the hang of this'! Now you do it without thinking.

If you have learned to drive a car, you will have gone through the same process. First, everything is done with conscious effort, and then suddenly there comes a moment when you are doing everything 'unconsciously'.

Oh! Just in case you don't wear lace-up shoes or drive a car. How about learning to brush your teeth?

So! Now you know that YOUR journey of "weight reduction and control" requires you to have an awareness and a desire for change and a commitment to:

Become the You – You will Become.

Look at yourself in the mirror – NOW,

At the start of this adventure, what do you see? Now, be gentle, but be honest as you look at yourself and describe to yourself the image you see.

Now imagine, as you stand in front of the mirror, that you are at a fairground arcade in the 'hall of mirrors'. You giggle as the mirror makes you appear fat, very fat, short, tall, and skinny. As you stand there, looking, the image changes and you find yourself standing in front of the 'look slim' mirror. See yourself, as you want to be wearing the type of clothes that you want to wear and in the colours you'd love to wear

Do that now! Use your imagination!

Remember? I asked you to do that in the 'Introduction'!

Now - hold that picture of the you, YOU want to be for a moment and remember it. Close your eyes and record it in your subconscious, because that will be one of the strategies you will use to achieve success. Open your eyes, and be on your way, doing whatever you now have to get on with.

That little exercise is called **'Visualisation' – Imagining – Imaging**.

The subconscious mind loves pictures and colours. Now, how easy was that?

So! Do it often. Once you've done it a few times you can just use the "mirror in your mind". Guess what it's called? – Imagination. Remember when you were growing up?

We have already come to the understanding that this process is a journey.

Know your starting point – know your finish point. Plan the steps to get from start to finish.

03

Next step.

Your body is unique and has all the information that you need to help you on your adventure. It is much, much smarter than you can imagine. The trouble is that we have lost the art of listening, whether to others or to our own bodies, or to the little small inner voice, called intuition – sometimes also 'gut feeling'.

Did you ever see the film 'The Dead Poets Society'? If you haven't, borrow it and enjoy the experience. In the film, Robin Williams as a newly arrived teacher takes his class into the hall and asks them to look at the school photos of all the previous students. And as they are looking, not knowing what they are supposed to see, he whispers: **"Carpe Diem." (Seize the Day).** He's asking them to imagine it's their graduation day.

The trouble with our society today is that there is so much noise and clamour. The mobile phone rings - the text message pings – the I pod does whatever they do, so we don't hear our body's important messages being passed to us. Sometimes the message clamours to be heard. At other times it's just a gentle whisper.

What's the relevance of that story? The body, controlled by the unconscious, is talking to us all the time but we choose, either, not to listen or we hear but ignore the advice we are being given. If you don't seize the day – the day will seize you.

If you don't listen – the moment is gone!

Picture this scene:

Father holding newspaper up in front of his face while reading it. Child, sitting on the floor asking questions and being ignored and just getting the cursory "Uhh". "Uhh" Eventually the child pulls the paper down and says. Will you listen to me with your FULL face".

Children have a delightful way of saying things – don't they?

Don't ignore the body's promptings. LISTEN and take NOTICE

The body will tell you when you are hungry and when you have had enough. Listen, and heed the message.

Trust your body. Trust your intuition. Then commit yourself to action.

Kinesiologists practice the therapeutic art of Kinesiology, which uses muscle testing to diagnose the body's diseases. They believe that they are more accurate in their diagnosing than doctors, because the body tells them the truth.

Learn to listen, to hear and to act on your body's signals. It will tell you when you are hungry and when you are thirsty.

That is really important. It's so obvious, but we ignore this inner wisdom.

Eat when you are hungry.

Many of us do not follow this simple rule and then pay the consequences. We ignore the fact that each of us is a unique individual and we each have a different metabolic structure.

We have all come into contact with people who seem to eat mountains of food and the 'wrong' types of 'goodies' and never put on weight. Then there are others, who only seem to 'look' at certain foods and they can't fit into clothes they wore "only yesterday"!

Many of us eat because we have established certain habit patterns that are not serving us well. Sometimes you will hear the cry, 'I'm hungry all the time'. Other times 'I'm never hungry', but they still eat! Strange, isn't it?

So! Make friends with your body and listen to its messages.

Isn't that what you do with friends – listen to them?

If you take this lifestyle on board you will be on the first step to breaking your 'dieting' regime and achieving a slimmer body, vibrant with health and energy.

When you starve yourself, by not eating, after you have received the hunger signals from your body, your body wants to store fat. So, if you have been dieting for some time, your body could be stuck in the 'fat storage' mode.

When you starve yourself, your body thinks a famine is coming and goes into survival mode and says to itself, "famine coming – store fat just in case it's needed", so it stores fat in your cells.

Many people say that they skip breakfast because they are not hungry! **This is NOT HELPFUL!**

We need to kick-start the metabolism & use the acid that is made by the stomach in anticipation of eating at the start of the day.

A habit is formed and the body goes into 'habit mode' and pinches fat from whatever foods you eat. So if you eat when you don't need it or just because "it's meal time" the body will grab and store fat for the anticipated famine.

We humans have our own storage places. Did you know that? Guess where? Generally, for a man it's in the stomach, and for a woman, in the hips and thighs!

Consistently ignoring your body's cries for food alters your metabolism. A faster metabolism burns more calories as you go through the day. When you stop yourself from eating when you are hungry, your metabolism slows down to allow your body to conserve energy, leading sometimes to lethargy or in some cases, a mild depression.

The flip side – oh yes, there is always a flip side – is, that if you don't eat when you are hungry it sets up dysfunctional patterns of thinking in the subconscious mind in connection with food. These misleading signals cause tensions and trigger powerful neuro-chemical changes in the brain, leading to false signals and perverse behaviour patterns – like cravings and bingeing.

A vicious cycle has been set in motion. The less you trust your body, the less trustworthy your body's messages become. Before you go into a downward spiral of despair, here's some good news.

Listen to your body, to reset the pattern of eating whenever you feel hungry. Within a few days of persevering, your metabolism will stabilize. Your body will establish new patterns of behaviour, taking nutrients only when it really needs it to support your needs of the moment, then, it will release the surplus.

Simple. Yes! Easy? Maybe? Take a moment to close your eyes.

See: "The You, You Wish To Be".

Wearing the colours you would love to wear

Remember the subconscious likes pictures and colours.

You could add movement – walking, dancing, gymnastics or singing.

Have fun!

Step 3: Eat What You Want - But - Be There!

Listen to your body and that will lead you to eat what you want, and not what you think you should eat. If you do that, listen to your body, you will begin to break habit patterns that have served you ill.

We have all heard of the strange and weird food cravings that many women have during pregnancy. Very often family members have great fun with that and ask, "Wow! Where did that come from"?

The answer to that is – 'her body'. The reason is that her body is telling her what it is deficient of and what it needs, to continue to do its job of 'baby building'. The cravings can vary from pickled onions to ice cream and perhaps even more strange requests.

Diets usually come with a list of do's and don'ts. The trouble is, that as soon as you are told, "Don't", it becomes forbidden fruit and in some strange way, more desirable. Now you are in conflict mode and that can be very wearing on your physical, nervous, spiritual and mental systems.

However, as soon as you begin to listen to your body, any tensions and guilt will evaporate. You will notice subtle changes in your desires and your taste buds will redefine your likes and dislikes.

Again, studies have proved that you won't end up on a diet of cakes, chocolate, pizzas, and burgers. Remember, your magical body will help you develop a natural attraction to other foods that are more beneficial for you – if you allow it to do so?

Now that we have looked at the "Eat what you want" strategy, let us look at the next step.

TIP 1   "Be there"

Be there. Be in the present moment.

Having worked with overweight people, one very strange idiosyncrasy has emerged. They spend a lot of their time thinking about food, except when they are actually eating it -Weird?

Then they almost shovel the food in to their mouths, without either chewing or tasting it? Now, why would they do that?

They know that to survive, they have to eat. What they are unaware of is, that any survival activity releases a chemical in our brains, called serotonin. This gives them a sort of 'high'. Sadly, their eating is 'unconscious', so they don't pick up their body's signal telling them, "I'm full. I've had enough". They continue eating, expanding their stomachs and putting on weight.

That temporary 'serotonin high' is followed by feelings of guilt. They feel so guilty that they repeat the whole sequence in order to anaesthetise the guilt feelings they have just created. And so it goes on.

Have you given second thoughts to how accommodating your body is? Once it realises that you are not listening to it and want to do your own thing, it goes into "flip" mode and will assist you. The skin stretches and stretches and stretches stealthily, without bursting. Like a Conifer – a sapling, then suddenly a GIANT.

Hush! - Listen! – be aware of the body's gentle signals!

Our adventure has truly started. This exciting strategy will help you change your habits so you can eat whatever you want. However, you have to be there to enjoy whatever it is you are eating in every single mouthful, as you chew - and enjoy the flavours of the food.

Another experiment showed that when people were blindfolded and were unable to see their food they ate about a quarter less. Why? Because, when they couldn't see, they found they concentrated on the taste and texture and were more open to the signals. They had blocked out the programming that said, "Don't leave any food on your plate – remember the starving children in some far distant part of the world." How could that ever help them?

Did You Know? There are restaurants where you eat in the dark.

You pre-order your meal. You are met at the door and led to your table in total darkness. The experience allows you to savour the flavour of your meal. I have a friend who has done, just to savour the experience.

Yes! You have to book a table, because they are so popular! Oh! and also very expensive. Isn't it wonderful you can do that at home for free?

Most of us have been programmed by well- meaning parents at some stage or another, with the command to clean our plates – "eat it all up – think of the starving children in some corner of the world." This subtle programming at a formative age, by people who were authority figures, will have left its mark, instilling a guilt factor into our psyches.

When one thinks about it, we wonder how this plate cleaning exercise could ever have helped the starving - anywhere?

Do you really think that cleaning your plate of excess food is going to prevent starvation elsewhere?

As a de-programming exercise try this and have fun with it.

TIP 2 Next time, just leave a little something on your plate. – it could be a potato chip or piece of vegetable and the subconscious will pick up the signal that you are making changes.

TIP 3   Use a smaller plate.

This will ensure you aren't tempted to over fill or over eat.

I have a theory - I could be way out, but it's a thought to ponder on.

Maybe restaurants and eating establishments give you big plates and too much food so as to allow them to justify the high charge. Maybe I'm wrong: it's just a thought. Many times a lot of food is left on the plate and is thrown away

When you last ate out – did everyone clean his or her plates?

Imagine this scene: The last time you went out in a mixed party –men and women - and you ordered your meals. Some would probably have ordered the same meal. Did you see the waiter/waitress making notes such as: 'One six foot guy, he'll need a lot. One skinny lady – give her less'? The reality is that both would have received the same size meal.

TIP 4   Sometimes, share a meal.

(I have experienced this in America, where it is considered totally acceptable to do so.)

TIP 5   For the next 21 days, slow your eating speed,

Chew each mouthful thoroughly and savour the flavours. It helps if put your cutlery down between each mouthful. This sends a signal to your conscious and subconscious minds that what you are doing is deliberate.

It gives your body time to notice the behaviour.

TIP 6   For picnics or finger buffets

Put your sandwich, or whatever you have chosen, down between each mouthful. When your mouth is empty, all you have to do is to repeat the process. This ensures that every bite is a conscious action and the shovel has been consigned to history.

Question? Have you ever wiped your plate clean at a restaurant, even though you were feeling "stuffed"? You had to finish every last morsel because you were committed to pay for it?

Another scenario! You are at friends for dinner. You are feeling full and don't really want any more but you are thinking, 'I can't leave anything, they'll think I don't like their cooking'!

Just as a matter of interest, "What did you do"?

Listen to your body! This is another interpretation of the saying, 'Listen to your gut feeling'. The more you tune in to your body's signals, the more noticeable they become. If you ignore the signals you will notice more and more discomfort if you continue.

Here is another interesting feature of your subconscious mind. Its primary function is to protect you, so it gives you signals to let you know if you are going off track.

NB. When people first start smoking, the signals are - choking, spluttering, coughing, foul taste, smell and acrid stinging. The flip side – yes, the flip side again – is, that when you choose to ignore the signals, the subconscious goes into 'Plan B' mode and says, 'I guess they want to ignore the 'primary care' signals and if smoking makes them happy, we can help them do that too'.

(It is always a source of psychological interest to me and others, that, smokers will walk up to the counter and say, "I'll have a packet of ..?" which clearly says, "smoking kills".

Your body is always giving you signals. Don't wait till you are either physically faint with hunger or ravenous. Because, as I said earlier, if you do, the body will start preparing for starvation and deprivation mode and you will end up eating more than you need, so that the body can store fat for later.

Eat when you feel the pangs of hunger. At first it may be a gentle nudge and then a slightly more insistent signal. The stopping point is, when you feel pleasantly satisfied or full.

In the early days you may stop too soon as your body is learning to interpret and understand the 'finish' signals. No problem! If the body tells you it needs food, eat, but only what you actually want or need, NOT what you think you should – subtle difference, but you'll get the hang of it.

There are various theories – it takes twenty-one days to change a habit; others say less - just be aware – be there - chew each mouthful thoroughly.

The real message is: Be there - Eat slower - Chew each mouthful with a conscious awareness, savouring the flavours.

Don't worry about the fact that others may have finished eating well before you. If they fret at having to wait for you to finish - that's their problem.

Another aside: Sometimes it's the mothers who develop the habit of eating fast, because they have babies and toddlers that may need instant attention.

However, if you are past that stage of caring for children, you can also change that unwanted habit too.

TIP 7   Forget The Scales

The daily weighing ritual. A word of caution: Forget the daily visits to the bathroom scales. That's an obsessive behaviour linked to the variety of diets that people are enticed to try.

Some people weigh themselves daily - maybe, morning and evening.

Some weigh after every meal, with high expectations. Checking daily is not an accurate way of monitoring. Each time you climb on the scales you are setting yourself up for a let-down. Everyone's weight fluctuates all the time, even slim people.

Why? Because your weight can fluctuate as much as ten pounds from environmental factors outside your control – atmospheric pressure and water retention. Slim people rarely weigh themselves.

Just focus on where you want to be and follow the guidelines outlined here — and you will get there. The strategies suggested will do the necessary tweaking and course corrections.

Consider an aircraft flying from one place to another, for instance, London to New York. It doesn't fly in a straight line. It's always adjusting its course to cater for variations in a number of factors, winds for instance.

It's said, that it could be off course about 90 percent of the time!

It's good to know that, because you will have some days that are better than others, with ups and downs that you will now take in your stride. Sometimes you will be buzzing with confidence about your 'weight reduction and control' programme and on other days, less so.

Focus on your goal and follow the strategies.

You will achieve your goal — YOU WILL SUCCEED

Success doesn't come to you — You go to it.

YOU WILL REDUCE YOUR WEIGHT and KEEP IT OFF.

You will feel better in your body, in your mind and in your levels of energy. Remember your image of yourself. Seeing yourself, daily, as you want to be, is better than any step up on to scales.

So, let's recap:

* You are on an adventure.

*You have developed new habits and attitudes.

*You have taken action and kept your focus on the end result.

Splendid! Terrific!

04

Put the kettle on and lose weight

Green tea is a great natural aid for weight loss.

Experts say that the substances present in green tea, help to inhibit the movement of glucose into fat cells.

Green tea may also act as a glucose regulator. It does this by slowing down the action of a particular digestive enzyme called amylase. This enzyme aids the breakdown of starches (carbs), which can cause blood sugar levels to soar following a meal.

It helps to slow the rise in blood sugar after a meal. This prevents high insulin spikes (lots of insulin promotes fat storage) and the subsequent fat storage.

The weight loss action performed by the green tea is by the way it maintains and lowers the blood sugar levels during meal times.

In other words, when green tea is included in your diet, your body isn't creating the substances which produce fat as readily as it normally would.

<div style="text-align: center">~~~</div>

Step 4: The Power of Imagination & Visualisation

We all have two minds – Our Conscious Mind and Our Sub-conscious (Unconscious) Mind, and each has its own attributes, idiosyncrasies and uses.

Willpower, part of our Conscious mind, has to be triggered each time you use it. Imagine going into a darkened room to get something or do something. You switch the light on, do or get what you want and as you leave you switch the light off. Willpower is like that. It does what you have asked it to do, and then it switches off and goes into "rest" mode till the next time you want to use it and switch it on.

Very often people say, "My willpower is good in this area of my life but not in that". The reality is that willpower has no 'choice making' or analytical capability - but we have. It simply means that we have chosen to use willpower in one situation and not in another.

If Willpower and Imagination are in 'competition', Imagination will always win. So it makes sense to use your imagination. The reality is that it is extremely difficult to break a habit using willpower alone, very simply, because habits are formed in the subconscious (unconscious) mind. **If you want to change a habit, that's where you have to go.**

You have probably tried willpower to help you in your dieting and been unsuccessful. Now you know the reason, don't beat yourself up. No guilt trips! There is a better way.

Use your IMAGINATION, and that is where the Subconscious Mind comes in. By way of reinforcement, remember it is in the Subconscious Mind that habits are formed and changed.

Let's go back to an earlier question. What is it that you want for yourself?

It is not in your interest just to say or think 'To lose weight' or 'I don't want to be fat' or 'To lose the fat around my thighs or my stomach'. Remember, you have to be specific. Remember your choice of words. If you 'lose' something you do your utmost to find it. Well! Don't you?

The image, thoughts and words you choose are so very important. They should always be personal, positive and in the present tense and that positive focus will give you results.

The subconscious only works in "THE NOW".

Did you look in the mirror this morning and see the image of the "You", you want to be, wearing the colours and clothes you want to wear?

If you didn't – why not? Too easy?

Be positive when you think and speak about what you want, then visualise/picture it, to be so. Whatever you focus on is what you will attract. That is the first rule of Psychology and the Law of Attraction. The subconscious will come to your aid and find a way. Conversely, the subconscious cannot understand and cope with the negative programme, 'I don't'.

You are what you eat for sure, but you are also what you think. So get used to thinking of yourself and seeing yourself as you wish to be – attractive - handsome – slim and the size you want to be – wearing the clothes and colours you'd like to wear.

In your bag of 'tools' you have two very powerful tools – Imagination and Visualisation, (Seeing Pictures in your Mind)

But - as with any tool, they are of no use unless you get them out of the tool box and use them as required.

Occasionally people say they cannot visualise. The truth is that everyone can visualise and we do it all the time. Sadly, sometimes when you give 'it' a label, people conjure up all manner of difficulties and problems. You may not have used this gift but it is still there within you, just waiting to be used.

Here's something to try for fun.

If I asked you to think of a horse, you would be able to picture a horse without any problem. If I asked you what colour it was, you would probably tell me without hesitation. Ask that question of a number of people and I'm sure that when you did a de-brief, you would find that we had horses of different heights, sizes and colours. Each one of us is unique but the gift is there for all to us.

If I asked you about your front door, with a little look inside your memory bank, you would be able to tell me what it looked like, what colour it was and where the handle was. Now, you would not be standing in front of your door physically, yet you had no problems seeing it in your mind's eye. That's all it is! Easy, isn't it?

Oh! And please, please don't think of a pink elephant!

Here's another game to play. It's simple and powerful.

If you decide to close your eyes, read through the following instructions before playing.

- Imagine you are sitting in a movie theatre. On the screen, you are watching a movie of yourself. You are having fun – doing whatever it is you have fun doing. You could be on a picnic, playing a sport, singing, dancing, or walking through the woods. It's your movie. You are the producer and director.

  In it you are slim, happy, having fun, full of confidence because you are seeing yourself as you aim to be, and feeling the emotions that go with that experience.

- Now! See that slimmer you doing all the things you normally do in your day-to-day activities and achieving them with ease. You see yourself eating just enough to satisfy your hunger. You see yourself refusing food or 'goodies' because you have had enough. You see yourself handling anything that comes your way with a new found emotional confidence.
- See how you carry yourself, talk to yourself, and move about as a slimmer, confident you would move.
- If the picture needs adjusting just adjust it. Imagine you have controls you can use to adjust the picture. Make it brighter. Make the colours more vibrant. Make whatever changes you want to make. You are in charge. You are the director and producer. Anything you don't like, either fade out or cut out. Imagine the cutting room floor littered with cuts you have made because they are no longer relevant to the story or the image you had in mind.

    It's your story. – It's your reality
- Run the movie again and view it with your new perspective. You have changed, grown in your perspective.

Repetition, Repetition, Repetition is the key to your success.

You can do this anywhere and no one needs know what you are up to.

Doing this anytime of the day and as often as you like, will make results come faster. Two very good times to run this film are first thing in the morning as you begin to emerge from sleep and again at night as you begin to drift into sleep.

The subconscious finds both these times especially receptive to your programming and desires.

However, you can do this at any time of the day and as often as you like. It only takes a moment or two, and no one needs to know what you are doing – play with it (Not while you are driving!!!!!)

Oh for the days, when as children we could 'daydream' whenever it took our fancy.

Life often leaves us with a sense of nervousness or excitement from time to time. Remember when you played hide and seek as a child? Wanting to be found, yet hoping you wouldn't be, while biting your nails with anticipation.

Here are some IMAGINATION thoughts to ponder on.

Until you give them meaning they are just words. Let them resonate within you.

> "You can't depend on your eyes when
> your imagination is out of focus."

> "Imagination has always had powers of
> resurrection that no science can match."

Did you know? Einstein and Thought Experiments.

Albert Einstein famously pictured himself travelling through space on a beam of light as a way to develop the theory of relativity. This may seem an odd way to solve a complex physics problem, yet he often used imaginary scenarios to understand the world and formulate his theories.

To encourage fresh thinking we can all benefit from 'daydreaming believing'.

Hold this thought: "If it worked for Einstein, it is working for me".

05

Step 5: Change your habits – Change your Life

Take a moment to look at some of your habits, both good ones and 'bad' ones. When you get to the 'bad' ones, don't go on any guilt trips. You are just looking!

Now jot down some habits you will change.

Then come back here and continue your adventure.

Few things are more difficult than kicking bad habits, or developing more positive ones, BUT, it is definitely worth the effort. Bad habits, like smoking, overeating or self-criticism, shorten lives and lead to under-achievement, and unsuccessful attempts to change them, lower our self- esteem.

In contrast, good habits create a kind of "success auto-pilot," leading to greater accomplishment with less thought and less effort. So how do you best eliminate bad habits and create good ones?

1. Replace a bad habit with a good one. Eliminating a habit is much harder than replacing it with a more productive habit. Studies of people who compulsively bite their fingernails have shown that it is difficult for them to completely give up their habit, but much easier for them to substitute biting with the more productive habit of grooming their nails.

2. Exercise. A habit of regular exercise is obviously important for lasting weight control. Exercise helps in eliminating a number of bad habits.

3. Reward Success. The most fundamental law in all of psychology is the "law of effect." It simply states that actions followed by rewards are strengthened. Unfortunately, studies show that people rarely use this technique when trying to change personal habits. Setting up formal or informal rewards for success, greatly increases your chances of transforming bad habits into good ones, and is far more effective than punishing yourself for bad habits or setbacks.

4. Schedule your bad habits. If you are struggling to kick a bad habit, perhaps limit the habit to a specific time and place. Research and case studies confirm that this rather unconventional approach can be a useful first step in changing bad habits. How is that for a Creative approach?

Points to think about:

No. 1 Excellence is a Habit. We learn by observation, imitation and repetition

No. 2 Habits are like submarines. They run silent and deep. First we make our habits, and then our habits make us.

Habits are like comfortable beds. They are easy to get into, but difficult to get out of.

Winning and Losing — both are learned habits.

Choose your habits:

Bad habits begin unconsciously, then, layer upon layer, through practice, they grow from cobwebs into cables that shackle and diminish our lives.

Within you lies the ability to change habits that no longer serve you. All you have to do, is to focus on what you want - **NOT on what you don't want.**

Let me repeat that.

Focus on what you want – NOT on what you don't want.

Vagueness confuses the unconscious mind. For instance, "I want to be slimmer", or "I want to weigh less". Reducing a pound or two would meet that target but that's not satisfactory if you want to get rid of a stone, or two, or more. Be specific about what you are aiming for.

Look at the habits you have developed. See if they serve you. If not, start replacing them. Yes! It will mean stepping out of comfort zones. Isn't that where the adventure lies and where growth and the rewards are?

Have fun. Imagine you are in the hall of mirrors and you are looking at the slim you.

Smile! Feel that glow of success.

06

Write down some of the habits you will change:

Habits work with all the precision of a marvellous computer.

To change anything you have to — TAKE ACTION

Step 6: The Emotional Roller Coaster.

One of the contributory factors to weight gain and obesity is the way we handle our emotions, so let's look at what we mean when we say "emotions" or "emotional."

Rub our Aladdin's Lamp of Language and the dictionary has this to say:

"Emotion": Agitation of the passions or sensibilities, often involving physiological changes. Any strong feelings, as of joy, sorrow, reverence, hate or love arising subjectively rather than through conscious mental effort - taking place within an individual's mind in a manner unrelated to external reality.

Did you notice that statement?

Taking place within an individual's mind in a manner unrelated to external reality.

Practically everyone, whom the dieting seesaw has enslaved, has confirmed that a huge part of his or her problem has been 'emotion related'. Having had that wonderful insight it has been hard to understand why they have still pursued dieting regimes, which take little or no account of resolving the emotional and psychological issues.

Unresolved emotional issues silence or confuse the body's signals that tell you 'I'm satisfied, and I've had enough'. We all know, that if you ask the wrong question you will rarely get the right answer.

People on diets are maybe asking the wrong question.

They generally ask, "What should I eat?"

In most cases the right question could be, "What's eating me?"

Please, don't confuse physical hunger with emotional hunger. Satisfying physical hunger will never resolve emotional hunger or vice versa.

You know how physical hunger works. It generally creeps up on you with a sort of light headedness, or you hear and feel your stomach rumbling or you have a gradual awareness that it's a long while since you ate. Once you have satisfied your physical hunger, you can be sure you will receive hunger signals a few hours later. Your energy boiler needs to be stoked.

- Emotional hunger is generally 'not gradual'.
- Once you have satisfied the emotional hunger it doesn't come back four or five hours later.
- Emotions are linked with feelings. Change the feelings you experience and you will change the emotions and their intensity.

Emotional hunger is very real, and will certainly reflect the many situations going on in your life. Usually, it is as a result of low self -esteem, feeling unloved, unappreciated, taken for granted, feeling worthless and helpless and often also due to something even harsher – self-loathing.

Uniquely, it's not something we share with others, so the more you focus on your self-loathing the more you feed it and it grows.

Story Time

There is the story of a young Native American boy who was disturbed about some of his behaviours and thoughts. He sought his grandfather's help and said, "Grandfather, sometimes I feel that I have two wolves fighting inside me and I am frightened that something terrible will happen. What can I do to make the bad wolf go away?" The grandfather looked at the boy with compassion and drawing on his wisdom, gently said, **"Which one do you feed?**

That is the story of our lives. Mind and Body are intertwined. We don't really need research to tell us that our thoughts have a significant effect on our health and well-being.

What are you thinking about yourself when you look into a mirror? "My thighs are huge – my arms and face are flabby– my buttocks are gross. I am obese – my face is wrinkled it looks like a prune"! I'm sure you can add to that!

Now, Supposing I walked up to you in the street and said "Wow! Your thighs and legs are huge. Your arms are a bit flabby and your buttocks are gross. You've been sitting on them a bit. All in all, you are sort of obese. Oh! By the way, your face has a few more wrinkles."

What would you do? Hazarding a guess, I'd say, I would most likely be picking myself off the street or be nursing a very sore face.

Yet! You do that do yourself again and again and just take it. Did you smile? I hope so!

You may not be religious or spiritual but I'd love you to consider these words of wisdom from the Bible. I'm sure other Spiritual Books will say something similar.

Here they are: **"Do unto others as you would have them do to you".**

Here's the flip side. You have to smile! There's always a flip side!

NLP, (Neuro Linguistic Programming) does the same thing by another name and that is called 're-framing'. So let's re-frame the Biblical saying.

Do unto yourself, as you would have others do to you.

Can you do that? I'm sure you can. **How much easier can it get?**

Story Time:

Are you sitting comfortably? Then I'll begin. First, however, let me apologise up front to you ladies who are reading this. It could easily apply to us men, but this is the way I received the story.

Ladies if you have a man in your life, who could take the man's place in this story, be gentle – please! I said "gentle"!

The wife is looking in the mirror and as she looks she says "My thighs and legs are huge. My arms are a bit flabby and my buttocks are gross. I've been sitting on them a bit. All in all, I'm sort of obese. Oh! By the way, my face has a few more wrinkles, looks a bit *pruney*".

Then she turns to her husband, who has been sitting on the edge of the bed watching this ritual, and says, "Honey, say something nice and positive to give me a lift".

{Poor Sucker} Realising he is now in a very difficult situation, he pauses for a moment to consider his response and comes out with this. "Darling! Your eyesight is perfect"!

I was never told how the story ended, so I'll leave you, (men and women) to ponder on that!

By the way did you laugh? Remember? "Laughter is the best medicine!"

It's true though! We are prepared to build others up, yet we find it so hard to do the same to ourselves.

Are you still wondering how that story ended???
Beware.

Careless thoughts and words will cost you the life you aspire to.

The thoughts You think -, is YOU talking to yourself!

There have been many research studies done on the subject of our thoughts. Some studies say, we have between 50,000-70,000 thoughts per day, which means between 35 to 50 thoughts per minute, per person.

What are you saying to yourself?

My mother's advice to us kids was, "Words are powerful. Use them wisely. They are like an arrow shot from a bow. Once released they cannot be recalled!"

Our thoughts and words are Powerful. They are Active and very Energetic. Used Unconsciously or with Disrespect, they bring Chaos.

Remember, your Subconscious, Unconscious mind is on 24 hour duty, day in and day out. It listens and takes on board what you focus on and will give you just that.

So, please, don't beat yourself up or take any guilt trips. It's not the merry-go-round to be on. Just take responsibility!

You and I are where we are, because of the choices and decisions we have made over our lifetime. Begin to see yourself with all the beautiful character traits you have kept under wraps. As you begin to see yourself, as you would love to be, it will begin to happen.

So, see yourself as lovable, efficient, capable, reliable and beautiful. The saying goes, "Beauty is in the eye of the beholder" and "You are the beholder"!

Beauty is not just outward physical beauty, but the inner beauty that has its own luminescence and inimitable way of shining through.

Nelson Mandela quoted this at his inaugural speech, when sworn in as the President of South Africa in 1994.

Let's go back to becoming slimmer.

WHO AM I?

Our deepest fear is not that we are inadequate.
Our deepest fear is that we are extremely powerful
It is our light, not our darkness that frightens us.
We ask ourselves, "Who am I to be Brilliant.
Or Gorgeous, Talented and Fabulous?"
Actually, who are you not to be?
You are a child of God!
It's not just in some of us; it's in everyone.
(Marianne Williamson)

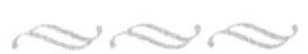

Apparently, less than one percent of women have the genetic potential to have what is reckoned as the 'model figure'. Each of us has a genetic blueprint and we at some stage or another have interfered with the natural design and shape of our bodies by doing things, eating inappropriately and not exercising in a way that is compatible with a healthy vibrant body.

You can only start where you are now and that begins with 'loving' the body you currently live in, so make peace with it. Thank it for having kept you alive and move on to making the changes for the slimmer, fitter, more vibrant and confident you.

(These techniques work with people who have eating disorders such as anorexia and bulimia. However, if you suspect or have been told that you are suffering from either, please seek advice from your doctor or other qualified professional.)

One of the challenges with anorexics and bulimics and indeed with many others is, that they only see or hear what they want to see or hear. (Perverse?)

Compliments and uplifting messages are filtered out. Their low self-esteem and low self-image filter out those messages, because they don't fit with who 'they think they are'.

Have you ever been told you look great and your response has been something like this "Oh? I just threw this dress on", or "I just put some lipstick on in a hurry ", or something similar for you men, such as "this shirt was a present" rather than just saying "Thank you"

How about when someone thanked you for doing a good job or making a great presentation? How often do we just accept the compliment and say, "Thank you"? More often than not we respond with a reply that diminishes the compliment. True or false?

Go back and read the poem - Who Am I - again.

Orange Juice

Picture an orange.

cut that orange in half and squeeze it. What comes out? The answer is 'Orange Juice'. Now! Why does orange juice come out when you squeeze an orange? The answer is.... because that's what's inside.

Correct!

Does it matter WHO squeezes the orange?

Does it matter WHERE you squeeze the orange?

Does it matter at WHAT TIME you squeeze the orange?

Of course not! Only orange juice will come out of an orange, because that's all that's inside an orange!

Now picture yourself. Imagine you're being squeezed–. Bills to be paid - kids to be cared for, your relationships are messy, you don't feel so good. You've gained a few extra pounds.

Squeeze: What comes out of you? Low Self Esteem, Anxiety, Stress, Anger, Rage, Doubt, etc. Why does Low Self Esteem, Anxiety, Stress, Anger, Rage or Doubt come out of you?.....because that's what's inside!

Does it matter who does the squeezing? Does it matter HOW tightly they squeezed? Does it matter HOW many times they squeezed or for HOW long?

Of course not! It couldn't come out if it weren't in you.

THE SOLUTION is: Don't BLAME people, circumstances and events for your fears and mood swings.. They are just showing you WHAT's INSIDE YOU.

It means, deep within, you're focusing on a LIFE you DONT WANT rather than **A LIFE YOU DO WANT**

Take control of your mind and actions NOW and your LIFE WILL CHANGE for the better. CHOOSE YOUR THOUGHTS, moment by moment if necessary. Do activities that make you smile and feel good. Talk to people who will make you laugh.

Anxiety is a natural human emotion, but worry accomplishes nothing, except to take away your emotional energy

And think of an orange OFTEN!!

BE HAPPY ---------------- DON'T WORRY

Everyone has a special place that holds a PEACEFUL memory.

EXHALE - then BREATHE IN GENTLY & VISIT IT IN YOUR MIND

Do it: – NOW.

07

Step 7: Exercise –Simple Steps to Keeping Fit.

Let's rub Aladdin's lamp and see what the dictionary says about Exercise.

"Activity that requires physical or mental exertion, especially when performed to develop or maintain fitness".

That exertion causes your heart to pump faster and you to breathe more deeply.

It doesn't say you have to pump iron or run marathons, but there is nothing to stop you, if that is what you would like to do. But, as with anything you want to do, it is better to follow a process. For someone to run marathons without training would be foolhardy.

Exercise burns calories and increases your 'basal metabolic rate'. That's the key -'the increase'. Basal metabolism is the least amount of energy required to maintain vital functions, such as respiration and digestion, in an organism at complete rest.

Are you a 'couch potato' with the television on?

Sometimes you might hear the myth "I cannot lose weight because I have a slow metabolism". So! You aren't a tree! Move, get the heart pumping and increase your metabolism. Your metabolism is not fixed, moored in concrete.

Make the decision and then implement that decision with action.

You are responsible for you! No one Else!

Exercise or sports may sometimes be painful and outside your comfort zone. Athletes push themselves to the limits to achieve better results. Consider Doctor Roger Bannister who, in May 1954, was the first person to run a mile under four minutes. He pushed his limits, knowing that all his knowledge and training and awareness had lead him to that moment in his life.

His motivation was that he had a goal! He wanted to run and achieve that four- minute mile. He ran it in just one second under. Small steps can start every journey

What is your GOAL?

Are you prepared to do what is necessary to achieve that goal? The steps we have outlined have been simple.

Do you remember step 3? I said, "BE THERE"!

Some suggestions to consider:

Swimming – Dancing – Gymnastics – Badminton – Tennis – Table Tennis – Squash –Skipping – Jogging (jogging on the roads is an impact activity that could lead to knee problems – so take advice on that) – an alternative is to use a "Bouncer" – (a mini trampoline, which can be used indoors and is easy on the knees) – Elliptical walkers - Yoga – Tai Chi

It's fun, it's easy, and it's safe for almost anybody of any age.

NASA stated, "the most efficient and effective exercise yet devised by man is Rebounding!

Put simply – bouncing on a mini trampoline. The aim isn't to bounce high or perform gymnastic tricks, but to perform a series of small, controlled movements.

Benefits of, which is a zero-impact exercise:_

- Improves circulation
- Increases the capacity of heart and lungs
- Lowers cholesterol levels
- Improves co-ordination and balance
- Reduces stress and tension
- Improves muscle tone (particularly legs, thighs, hips, abdomen and arms)
- Increases energy and vitality
- Boosts the lymphatic and immune system
- Fits in with your lifestyle
- AND IS GREAT FUN!
- Plus, unlike many other aerobic activities, rebounding places no strain on the joints of your body

Who Can Rebound?

It's very good for people who may have a knee injury and can't run on the ground for any distance. Put on a good CD and bounce along. Its great exercise

Mums, dads, children, grandparents… Rebounding is suitable for all ages and abilities! Stabilizing bars can be fitted which may help if you feel unsteady or are elderly, disabled or handicapped.

08

Stepping Stone 8: The Elixir of Life

The Miracle Liquid that cuts heart disease, helps us lose weight, and beats cancer.

There is a miracle cure on tap in your own home, right now, and it's cheap. There is no need to dash to the supermarket and load your car with heavy expensive bottles. This colourless liquid helps combat the risk of heart disease and many cancers and, yes; it can also help you lose weight.

So what is this wonderful cure?==== **WATER.**

Did you know that about 70% of our body weight is water, and it is vital for the efficient functioning of every cell in our body?

We know we can survive for several weeks without food, but only about three to four days without water. There is enough evidence to show that prolonged mild dehydration can lead to serious health problems. When you begin to feel thirsty, you are already showing signs of dehydration.

The British Dietetic Association says that adults should drink about 2.5 litres, (about five pints) of fluids a day; however, with normal functioning kidneys this is maybe unnecessary. Food provides about a litre a day.

If there any concerns consult your GP

The accepted suggestion is about six to eight glasses of water a day. Fruit juices, squash, weak tea and coffee help, but there are hidden dangers as a result of the processes they go through to bring them to the market place.

So WHY is it that we do, like the Ancient Mariner, paraphrase and say "Water, Water everywhere and not a drop we drink".

Some of the excuses we hear are so weak, one has to smile!

Don't like the taste — That's too much water to drink!

Yet we will drink pints and half pints of lagers and beers.

So for those who need a little help, here is a tip - carry a sports bottle, (of course any bottle will do) of water, preferably tap water, and sip from it as you go through your day.

Here are some thoughts to set you on your way. With the advances in knowledge and science these findings are ever changing, but they do give you an insight into how important water is to our wellbeing.

- Research, in America, found that people who drank four or more glasses of water a day, were less likely to get colon cancer than those who drank one glass or less. One theory is that drinking plenty of fluids dilutes possible carcinogens and pushes food through the digestive system more rapidly. (i.e.—minimises the time our 'stools' are in contact with the bowel wall)

- Not quite a "Fountain of Youth", but a water fountain, comes very close. The look of our skin is determined by its elasticity and the thickness of the dermis, that's the layer under the surface.

- About 50 percent of the dermis is water and dehydration makes it look dry, loose and prone to wrinkles. The British Journal of Dermatology published a study and its findings were that dehydration makes the dermis thinner, another sign of aging. Skin on the face was the most badly affected.

Another benefit of drinking plenty of fluids is that it reduces the risk of dementia in old age. It seems that a prolonged lack of water damages parts of the brain responsible for cognitive thinking.

- An American study found that drinking five glasses of water a day cut the risk of a fatal heart attack by 40 percent. One factor may be that the blood becomes slightly thicker when we are dehydrated ·

  * * *Dehydration is also a common cause of cramp. Gallstones, painful clusters- cholesterol, which can build up in the gall bladder, are more common in people who do not drink much water. A diet, high in fat and refined sugars, also increases the risk of gallstones.

- WOMEN, apparently can reduce their risk of breast cancer by as much as 79 percent by drinking five or more glasses of water a day. Women who have been through the menopause obtain the greatest benefit. It's believed that mild dehydration affects the enzymes within cells that clear toxins from the body.

  A rumbling tummy can be a sign of mild dehydration. Having a drink, when you think you want a snack, can help you shed pounds. Dehydration can also fuel cravings for junk foods.

  WATER - drunk before meals, reduces overeating

- Professor Frank Cerny headed a study at Buffalo University in America to see what effect dehydration had on asthmatics, and he said, "Asthmatics are more sensitive to dehydration, but the reasons are not clear. Dehydration increases the risk of asthma attacks brought on by exercise. If you have asthma, dehydration may make it worse. By dehydrating yourself the airways also become dehydrated."

- Children should drink six to eight glasses a day – but boys over 14 need around 11. Studies have shown that people who are even slightly dehydrated do worse in tests of short-term memory, concentration and maths. Another study showed that if someone was thirsty, drinking a glass of water boosted performance on mental tests.
- Some warning signs could include nausea and dark urine.
- Another study published in the New England Journal of Medicine, found that drinking more than two litres of water a day halves the risk of bladder cancer. One theory is that drinking fluids flushes out cancer causing toxins.

So why is it that we ignore the body's many cries for water yet still persist with the habitual mantra: "Water, Water everywhere and not a drop we drink"!

NB: Water is a key component to life. No living creature can survive without a fresh supply of pure water each and every day.

If you do not consume enough fresh water every day, your body:

- will age faster
- appear fatter
- be more susceptible to germs and colds
- lose joint mobility
- and much more.

Generally Speaking

1. Most people who weigh less than 150 pounds require no less than 8-10 glasses per day.
2. Those who weigh between 150-250 pounds may require about 16 glasses per day.

NB: Remember, we are all unique individuals, so the information given here is a very broad generalisation. (If you have any concerns, consult your Doctor)

There will always be discussions and alternative views of almost anything and questions galore. The answers may vary from Consultant to Consultant.

Below is the answer, from a Cardiac Specialist to someone's question.

Are certain times of the day more beneficial, for drinking water?

Drinking water at a certain time maximizes its effectiveness on the body:

2 glasses of water after waking up - helps activate internal organs

1 glass of water 30 minutes before a meal - helps digestion

1 glass of water before taking a bath - helps lower blood pressure

1 glass of water before going to bed - avoids stroke or heart attack

Water at bed time will also help prevent night time leg cramps. Your leg muscles are seeking hydration when they cramp and wake you up.

09

Stepping Stone 9: The Breath of Life.

Some of these exercises can be done at any time and anywhere. Other's need more time and focus.

Conscious Breathing & Unconscious Breathing

Breathing is automatic and essential to your life, yet most of us do not breathe properly. This can be caused by poor posture, stress, or a lack of exercise, to name just a few possibilities. Breathing incorrectly depletes your oxygen levels, taxes your immune system, decreases energy, and allows toxins to accumulate in your body.

Chest breathers, only bring oxygen in to the top of the lungs, where the blood level is minimal and the flow is only about a tenth of a litre a minute.

Abdominal breathers take the oxygen to the bottom of the lungs where the blood is at its maximum and the flow is over a litre a minute.

The anatomical reason is that when man first got on to his hind legs to walk - the anatomical changes took place based on the simple law of gravity.

So, how do you know if you are breathing properly?

Place one hand on your abdomen and the other on your chest. Take a breath - and notice if your abdomen or your chest expands. If you feel your chest rise, you are breathing improperly. Proper breathing should take place in the abdomen. (Commonly known as Abdominal Breathing).

Use these simple exercises to correct poor breathing habits:

1. Expel air from your lungs first — then start the breathing exercises Take a slow, steady, deep inhalation through your nose, allowing your abdomen to expand. Then slowly expel all the air from your lungs. Do this a few times a day.

   You will be amazed at how it will relieve tension, increase your energy, and generate feelings of well-being. On the in- breath, start exhaling before you get to the peak of the in – breath. On the exhale – start the in breath before the exhale is exhausted.

Keep the rhythm relaxed and continuous

- Each time you exhale imagine you are clearing the sinus and letting go of any tensions.
- Do this exercise for six long breaths at least - or as many times as is comfortable. This is simply to indicate that you should give time to this and other breathing exercises.

10

Stepping Stone 10: The Magic Garden – that is our Mind

Even this garden needs tending and nurturing or the WEEDS will surely take over.

Every day is a new beginning
All of your yesterdays ended last night
It makes no difference how long you've been alive
They're all ended
This day is absolutely NEW— You have never lived it before

WHAT AN OPPORTUNITY - A New Day

Do not wait; the time will never be "just right." Start where you are.

Here are some tips to help keep your MIND garden well - tended and weed free!

1. Make Your Plan: Know where you are and where you want to be. Where will you start? What (tools) will you need to implement that plan? It is important to realise that 'Yesterday' has gone. It cannot be repeated or improved. 'Tomorrow', which is where you are

hoping to be, will be SHAPED by what you do now, Today.

2. Be TRUE to Yourself: Accept the way you are now. Accept that you are not perfect – no one is. Aiming for perfection leaves us 'not trying' and so setting ourselves up for continual disappointment. A person who considers themselves "perfect" is seen as a "pain in the neck" by others! (There is ALWAYS a flip side)

    Aiming for EXCELLENCE is an achievable target. Even someone you admire will have their shortcomings – a fact!

    Michael J Fox, put it this way, "I'll do my best while striving for excellence. Perfection? I'll leave that to God".

3. Build a support team you can trust: There are too many people who will try / want to jeopardise your mission. They are the 'naysayers' – "What makes you think you can do that"? So, you don't have a go. Whatever you do you will get a result. That result will give you feedback which is vital for 'learning'

www.ingramcontent.com/pod-product-compliance
Lightning Source LLC
Chambersburg PA
CBHW031420250726
48656CB00002B/752